HERBS FOR INDIGESTION

Acidity is a 'stress' condition which can appear as indigestion, ulcers, rheumatic and arthritic complaints, skin disorders and some forms of cystitis. The herbs recommended in this book have been selected for their success in alleviating these ailments, because of their different alkalising sedative, tonic, or blood-purifying properties.

HERBS FOR INDIGESTION

by

CERES

Drawings by Alison Ross

THORSONS PUBLISHERS LIMITED
Wellingborough, Northamptonshire

First published as
Herbs for Acidity and Gastric Ulcers 1976
This Edition 1981

ISBN 0 7225 0739 9

Printed and bound in Great Britain by
Richard Clay (The Chaucer Press) Limited,
Bungay, Suffolk.

CONTENTS

INTRODUCTION

Acidity is a vague and popular term, not altogether approved by the medical profession, but the state is none the less very real to the thousands who suffer various tiresome maladies that appear to be caused by it. There is no consolation in realizing that the causes of this state are not yet fully understood.

What acidity actually comes down to is that the reaction of the blood and other secretions are less alkaline, or more strongly acid, than normal.

It is the effort to correct this balance and achieve a normal state, that those with a tendency towards rheumatic and arthritic complaints, as well as many who suffer from occasional acute skin disorders and some forms of cystitis, are engaged in all the time.

The cause of gastric ulcers, too, is not fully understood but it seems likely that the chief of them is the inability of the mucous membrane which lines the stomach to cope, in certain conditions, with an excess of the essentially acid digestive juices.

All forms of stress, anxiety, worry, disappointment, fear, fatigue, excitement and even chilling of the system, which can stimulate outpourings of the hydrochloric acid and other gastric juices, should be avoided as far as is possible.

Whatever the cause, gastric ulcers are a very

serious symptom and those who suffer from them have to be under medical supervision, for there is no knowing when and if they may get worse.

Orthodox medicine seems only capable of palliating the condition with alkalizers, pain-killers and tranquillizers. But there is nothing to hinder those who want to help themselves from telling their doctors that they would also like to consult qualified 'unorthodox' medical practitioners, like herbalists, homoeopaths or naturopaths.

All practitioners will agree that the patient needs plenty of calm, rest, and small, easily digestible meals at shorter intervals, instead of the usual three big meals each day, as the condition appears to be aggravated when the stomach is empty.

Where there is any conflict of opinion shown at all it is likely to be in suggested diets, but, if these are to be tried, they must be introduced very gradually indeed so that orthodox diets and medicines are only supplanted very slowly. Any quick or sudden changes may do far more harm than good.

Many 'over acid patients are highly strung and the achievement of a more peaceful outlook is a definite step back onto the road to improved health. The practice of yoga is a great help in this respect since it permits sufferers to develop an ability to relax. Sadly it is not always easy to do this, but with a positive outlook on life it is possible to try other ways of self-help. Much can be done with the use of natural remedies and a start can be made with herbal teas that are physically and mentally soothing.

SEDATIVE DRINKS
Passion-flower tea, for example, exerts a gentle sedative effect, from which natural sleep follows

easily. Some herbalists include (or prefer) Skullcap to make a calming night or day drink. They will also recommend between-meal drinks of Barley-water, or Brown Rice 'milk' (made by washing thoroughly cooked rice in a little water and keeping all the liquid to drink). For thicker drinks, this particular 'milk' can be made from ground or 'creamed' Brown Rice, or indeed from finely ground, compost-grown oats or the famous Slippery Elm.

There are plenty of herbs to help acidity and in fact it has been difficult to restrict the selection for this book, but the author has chosen those which she and her family have found to be helpful.

Deep breathing, if correctly done, is usually beneficial, but the air which is taken in should be fresh! Many people who find that they occasionally suffer from acidity are better when they are on holiday and out in the open air more than usual. Anything, of course, that promotes relaxation is good.

There are a few more golden rules to help everyone. Alcohol and vinegar and citrus fruits – oranges, lemons and grapefruit – as well as rhubarb and spinach, should be given up entirely. White sugar and white flour should also be totally dispensed with! A little Barbados sugar or honey should be used when sweetening cannot be done without and finely-milled compost-grown wholewheat flour used for all home cooking.

Individuals vary a lot in their ability to assimilate different fruits and vegetables without increasing their acidity and the only way to find out what you can take is by trying out small quantities of juiced vegetables and fruit very gently with other bland foods.

Forget all about the frying-pan and avoid rich foods, especially any that are fatty or greasy. Change over by degrees to using unsaturated fats and if necessary use sesame salt for flavouring. Totally vegetarian diets help some people, others are loath to give up a little meat, fish and fowl. Grain and pulse diets, on macrobiotic lines, do wonders for quite a lot of 'over-acid' people.

But, once more, it is important not to rush anything at all – except an increase of proper, relaxed rest. Patience is essential, for nothing can be cured quickly, although the determination to chew all food more and more, so that the process of digestion starts in the mouth and the food goes down to the stomach in a softened moistened state, can do much to relieve discomfort and induce calmness. Think of the peaceful atmosphere of a cow sitting and chewing the cud and try to take more time for quiet meals!

Finally try out some herbal teas, like Mint or Maté instead of the usual Indian, Ceylon or China tea which can undoubtedly be improved upon, healthwise. Start drinking Dandelion coffee instead of the better-known pure Coffee-berry beverages, and persevere with it even if you don't like it as first. Above all, do not let anyone at all deter you from trying to lead a gentler, quieter, possibly more self-sufficient life in which your outlook is fixed on acquiring a calm spirit!

1

AGRIMONY
(Agrimonia eupatoria)

Agrimony is a tall perennial and common wild flower in Britain. It grows in hedgerows, or at the edges of woods and has a slender spire of small yellow flowers, hence its commonest country name of 'Church Steeples'. It is also sometimes called 'Cocklebur' and 'Sticklewort', both of which names must have come into popular use because the plant's bell-shaped fruits are ringed by a fringe of hooks. These hooks catch in the passer-by's clothing, or indeed, in animals' fur.

The whole plant smells faintly of apricots and is an old country remedy for a variety of maladies. Part of its Latin name was derived from the Greek *Argemone*, a word used for herbs that helped the eyes, and the rest from Mithridates Eupator, a king of ancient times who was very skilled in the uses of herbs as medicine. There are endless references, through the years, about the benefits that Agrimony confers on its takers.

The French used it as a drink to help sprains and bruises and it was named *Eau de Arquebusade* in the fifteenth century when Philip de Commines referred to its values in the Battle of Morat.

Until the end of last century, country people drank a tea made from fresh or dried Agrimony plant to help their rheumatism, or 'the screws', which is a slight indication of its uses for 'those of acid constitution'. Paracelsus recommended it, centuries ago, to be steeped in hot water to make

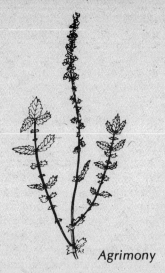

Agrimony

a footbath for tired feet. The herb was once included in the London Materia Medica, but it is not one of the 'official' herbs now.

A Victorian botanist gives it further praise by saying: 'The Agrimony is an ingredient in most of the herb teas which have been, from time to time, recommended', and it wins its place in this book about herbs to help acidity and gastric ulcers because it is a good safe stomach tonic which helps in the assimilation of food.

Agrimony also tones up a weakened or impaired digestion. It has a healing effect on any inflammation, both internal and external, and helps to get rid of feverish colds and general minor upsets. It is also said to be a blood-purifier; it was always included as an ingredient of yearly spring drinks and still seems to live up to its reputation of being a cleanser of the breath.

This plant could be said to be a panacea for so many small ills. It has other uses as well for the whole herb makes a good yellow dye. In the Tyrol it was considered to be a magic herb if it was drunk frequently enough because it was then said to give the sight necessary to be able to detect a witch in any guise! But in all seriousness again, it is one of the chosen healing herbs of Dr Bach, a modern qualified doctor and something of a magic healer himself.

2.

BALM
(Melissa officinalis)

Balm must be one of the most popular herbs of all time. It is on the 'official' list (see the Introduction to my *Herbs for First-aid and Minor Ailments* for an explanation of this term), and is a far too successful spreader in some gardens.

The plant's heart-shaped, deeply veined and crinkled leaves are aromatic (indeed the herb is sometimes called 'Lemon Balm'), and they are useful for culinary and medicinal purposes. Balm must, though, be kept under control, or it will invade every inch of the garden.

Balm is not a native of Britain even though it does so well in places here, but it has been popular, especially with bee-keepers, in this country. The Roman writer, Pliny, maintained: 'When bees have strayed away they do find their way home by it'.

For herbal uses Balm should be cut before it flowers, when the leaves are at their most aromatic. Used fresh, these leaves make a fragrant tea or *tisane*, but as the plant dies back in the winter, some should be gathered and carefully dried.

Culpeper said that it was 'an herb of Jupiter and under Cancer strengthens nature in all its actions'. Gerard was more specific, saying that 'it is good for those who cannot take breath unless they hold their necks upright'. He also extolled its virtues for students, because he stated that 'by a special

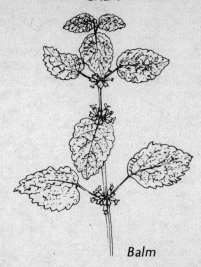

Balm

property it driveth away heaviness of mind, sharpeneth the understanding and increaseth memory'.

Certainly Balm tea has many uses. It can be made by pouring boiling water onto three or four leaves in a cup and is a most refreshing summer drink that is improved by the addition of a little honey and even by including an odd leaf of mint or fennel. It is cooling, whether iced or not, relaxing to a great extent, and good for the digestion.

Old Carmelite Water, 'spirit' of Balm, combined with lemon peel, Nutmeg and Angelica root, was drunk daily by the Emperor Charles V, as well as by the commoner John Hussey of Sydenham, near London, who lived to be 116 after breakfasting for fifty years on 'Balm Tea, sweetened with honey'.

A Welsh prince, Llewelyn, drank it every morning too, but only reached the age of 108.

The value of Balm for inflamed internal membranes lies in the fact that it is so 'kind to the stomach' and it is included here because it is easily found in many gardens. It is said to relieve depression, especially that which always seems to be associated with acidity, as well as being a safe carminative (dispeller or inhibitor of gas formation).

3.

BARLEY, BROWN RICE
and other Grains

Vegetarians and those who live on a more or less macrobiotic diet use grains a great deal to help provide nutrients that less unorthodox people probably take from the quantity of meat that they eat. Grains also, of course, provide bulk and roughage to help the digestion and the elimination of waste matter from the intestines.

Modern refined 'white' flour and cereals have always been depleted before they reach our stomachs and the advantages to everyone of using whole grains cannot be over-estimated. However, care is needed for sufferers from gastric ulcers and well-cooked Barley grains, without their husks, are recommended.

Barley is used, too, for making the famous soothing Barley Water, which (if uncontaminated by sugar and saccharine additives) is a safe drink for everyone although lemon, for those who are 'acid', should not be used to improve its flavour.

Brown rice, provided that it is repeatedly washed to remove loose husks before it is cooked, makes a far less acid-forming food than potatoes, and rice 'milk' from boiled ground rice is nourishing and useful as a between-meals drink. Brown rice, which is far richer in proteins than white or polished rice, is almost free of unsaturated fats and as long as it is chewed well in the mouth, as all food should be, before swallowing, it makes a most helpful addition to

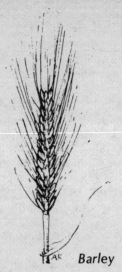

Barley

diets for everyone.

Maize, or corn, is not recommended for those with 'tender' stomachs, unless it can be picked very young and fresh 'on the cob' and cooked until it is soft. Tinned 'corn' seems to be difficult to digest at all times, unless it is masticated to pulp in the mouth. As it is often sweetened in the process of being tinned, those who suffer from acidity are advised to avoid it.

Other grains are usable in cooking, including Oats (see page 56), Buckwheat (which should be sieved after cooking, then pounded and flavoured with herbs), and, of course, Wheat from which bread, biscuits and cakes are baked. If it is possible to obtain compost-grown, finely milled and hand-milled wholewheat, this is always best, but however finely it has been ground, food made with wheat needs very careful mastication so that the digestive juices have already started their work on them in the mouth before they are received into the stomach.

It seems as if it is good advice for all those who are subject to acidity, to eat less than your luckier, more alkaline friends! Or perhaps it is better to say – less at a time! And this is especially true in the case of grain foods.

4.

CARROT
(Daucus carota)
and other vegetables

It is vegetables, primarily, and of course fruit, that provide our systems with vitamins and many essential trace elements. People who have a tendency towards acidity, and particularly those with inflammation of the lining of the stomach, may find cooked vegetables difficult to digest and accordingly may give them up in despair.

Before doing this, try very small quantities of raw vegetable juices, starting with the extremely beneficial carrot juice. The carrots need to be fresh, red, and – of course – clean – before being juiced but even a teaspoonful, at intervals during the day, can be a help.

Once it has been proved that this Carrot juice provokes no pain at all (and there is no reason why it should do so, even if it has to be taken with other light foods), an equally small quantity of finely grated, whole carrot root can be tried. Sesame salt, and sesame or sunflower oils can be added sparsely for flavouring and palateability by those who are unused to eating raw vegetables.

Cabbage juice, tried out in the same way, is a superb healer. The cabbage needs to be chosen for its youth, greenness and – again – freshness. Of course, preferably all vegetables should be compost-grown, out of the garden, and free from any taint of toxic pesticides and weed-killers.

Many 'stomach sufferers' eschew cauliflowers completely, finding them flatulent, apart from

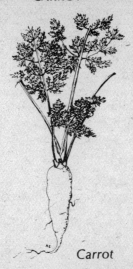

Carrot

anything else. But in small quantities they can be digested far more easily raw than cooked. Remember, too, that cooking has other disadvantages in that it kills, or partially kills, most of all plants' vitamin contents.

By careful and patient experimenting, the diets of those in whom unwanted acid conditions are only too easily encouraged can be slowly enlarged and made more interesting by the addition of far more fresh vegetable and salad plants than they would ever have dared to hope for.

Avocado Pears, eaten without dressings, make splendid fresh food for almost anyone except, perhaps, those with active gastric ulcers – but even the latter could try a minute quantity of bland green, ripe Avocado pulp with other food, or gruels.

There are, in fact, only a few raw vegetable plant foods that seem to the author to invite trouble. These include Spinach, Rhubarb, Green

Peppers and Tomatoes. Vinegar, of course, as has been stated elsewhere in this book, should be avoided like the plague! So, in the majority of cases, should Turnips, Swedes and Parsnips, but the occasional Radish, and even a little fresh, undressed cooked Beetroot are tolerated by some sufferers, while Lettuce, Watercress, and Corn-salad, if introduced gradually, are all usually 'safe'.

5.

CELERY
(Apium graveolens)

Celery is now imported into Britain from many other countries to supplement our home-grown crops. It is a useful culinary and salad vegetable and has antacid properties as well.

Wild Celery, or 'Smallage' or 'Ache', to give it two of its old popular names, grows by the sea in Britain and has dark green shiny leaves, always said to be poisonous. Cattle leave them severely alone, but it is an attractive plant to find, and if it is picked or bruised, it smells very strongly of the garden Celery with which we are more familiar.

A Victorian horticulturalist wrote: 'Garden Celery is rendered wholesome by bleaching but mere loss of colour is not the only consequence of plants being kept in the dark. Poisons, when it is the nature of the plant to yield poisons, are all formed in leaves by the action of light; the absence of this wonderful agent will therefore prevent the formation of poisons, as well as the formation of colour; and hence blanching renders the poisonous plant harmless.'

As this seems to be considered still correct, and as there is a certain amount of green Celery often on sale, a more modern scientific opinion was sought. Sir Edward Salisbury, a retired Director of the Royal Botanic Gardens at Kew in Surrey was asked his opinion and he answered that the above reasoning was far too sweeping. 'Blanching', he maintains, 'would never make such poisonous

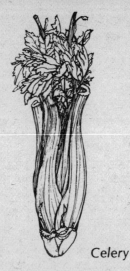

Celery

plants as Deadly Nightshade harmless, although it is possible that it may have had that effect, eventually, on wild Celery. Nowadays, the different strains of cultivated Celery have probably become altogether non-toxic and are therefore safe to eat, whether white or pale green.'

Blanched Celery always seems to have a better flavour, but this may be nothing to do with its colour, or even people's psychological reaction to an old favourite. It could be simply due to different soil, climate, and methods of cultivation.

It is interesting that Celery, used as a herbal remedy, fulfils the need for a digestive, especially if it is eaten at the end of a large, rich meal when discomfort and some distension seem to be almost inevitable.

It has the reputation of being an antacid in its own right, as well as an appetite-restorer and a nerve-steadier. Some herbalists credit it with the power of helping those with high blood-pressure and say it can also be used to improve 'tired' sight. Celery can be juiced, or, if necessary, very finely grated.

Celery seeds are good for heartburn; for sleeplessness, even for depression, as well as for helping those who have a dry tickling cough or an insatiable craving for apples! They should be used in these cases to make a herbal tea or *tisane*.

6

CHAMOMILE
(*Matricaria chamomilla* and or *Anthemis nobilis*)

There are two Chamomiles used by herbalists. The first is usually called German Chamomile (*Matricaria chamomilla*) but can also be found under 'True' Chamomile, or 'Hippocrates Chamomile', and the other is the English, Common, Roman or Belgian Chamomile (*Anthemis nobilis*).

There is not much difference in their superficial appearances for both have daisy-like flowers, with white outer ray florets and a cushion of golden disc florets in the centre. It means, unless people have good botanical experience, that they and other members of their 'family' can be difficult to identify, which is one reason for buying the herbs you use medicinally from reputable herbalists. It is also a reason for learning their Latin, or scientific names.

There is some difference in the medicinal uses of the two Chamomiles too. Both are soothing herbs for the stomach, but each suits patients of different temperaments!

German Chamomile is helpful for choleric, quick-to-anger sufferers from indigestion, 'soreness of the belly', or wind, and anyone who is impatient to the point of being irritable can benefit from taking this herb. It is splendid for fretful babies when they are teething. One of the indications, indeed, for its use is when anyone, including very young children, has one flushed and one pale cheek.

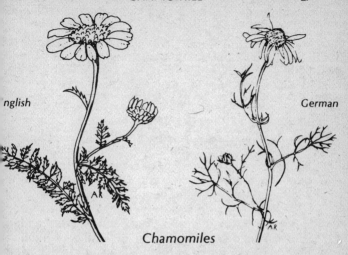

Chamomiles

A tea made from German Chamomile helps anyone with tooth or gum ache and it also alleviates heart burn and nausea, especially if it is worse after drinking coffee. Herbalists have used this plant for centuries for those with 'acid risings', a bitter taste in the mouth, and 'to dispel the wind loudly from those who need to lose it'.

The same plant is a useful and mild sedative and helps to 'quieten them who be restless' as well as peevish. It really is a useful herb for those that are difficult to live with and enables them to become less 'prickly'.

English Chamomile (*Anthemis nobilis*), used for planting fragrant, even if tough lawns, on one of which Sir Francis Drake was supposed to be playing bowls when the Spanish Armada was sighted, helps people with calmer temperaments in much the same ways, particularly if they are suffering from 'hot' or 'burning' indigestion or need a mild stomach tonic. It is also useful as a 'herbal tea' for inducing sleep to 'them who toss and turn'.

7.

COMFREY
(Symphytum officinale)

Some years ago there was a fashion for growing a blue-flowered, tall, cultivated Russian Comfrey as a forage crop which could also be used as excellent green manure. Some plants of this species still linger in the British countryside and tower over the common native Comfrey, which has only dingy white or purple flowers.

Comfrey is famous because it is thought to have the power of helping to knit together bones that have been fractured. In the old days fractures were surrounded by a poultice of its big hairy leaves instead of one made with plaster of Paris. As the leaves were put on, layer over layer, they set and hardened to form an external splint and their medicinal virtues could be absorbed through the patient's skin.

The whole plant is also full of mucilage. If the leaves are boiled as a vegetable, their hairiness disappears and they become slimy; it is this soothing mucilaginous property which makes the herb useful to those who need demulcent drinks. Some people seethe a few Comfrey leaves in Barley water to add to its thin, gruel-like consistency.

Comfrey tea helps all kinds of colds and coughs as well as bronchitis and even asthma sufferers have claimed that it has improved their condition.

The plant is less acid than Spinach or Beet and the leaf, or actually the whole plant, is said to be

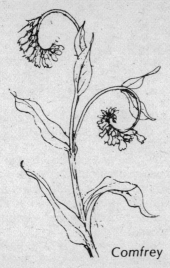

Comfrey

rich in vitamin B12, the only one of our wild plants at the time of writing that is known to contain it. Comfrey, therefore, can augment diets that are deficient in B12.

It is B12 that vegetarians and vegans find so difficult to obtain naturally; it is usually given to those who need it badly in the form of an extract from animals' livers.

Comfrey fritters, for those who feel it safe to eat lightly fried foods, are delicious if a few young leaves are dipped in a thickish, wholemeal flour batter and then cooked on both sides.

8.

CORIANDER
(Coriandrum sativum)

Before the days of clean cereal crops, when red poppies, corn marigolds and even a few cornflowers used to colour the big fields, Coriander was occasionally found as an 'escape' among seed that must have been imported from warmer climates.

It is a frail, faintly pink-flowered little umbelliferous plant which, when its fruits ripen, produces round, very flavoursome seeds.

Coriander can be grown in gardens in Britain, but it is difficult to get ripe seeds from the plants unless there is a hot, sunny summer, and they never seem to smell as unpleasant here as they do when they come from hotter climates.

The name Coriander is derived from the Greek 'koris' – which means 'a bug' – and the seeds when first gathered were once thought to 'stink of bugs'. They provide, however, quite a different and pleasant smell once they are dried and give a distinctive, interesting flavour to mixed spices. They are also used to flavour liqueurs. Actually a modern herbalist likens the scent of them to oranges!

The plant has been used since pre-historic times and the first records of it appear in Ancient Egyptian stone carvings. It was considered important enough to be cultivated commercially here during World War II and during those years it was found to be difficult to harvest it without its

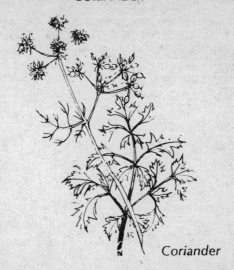

Coriander

pill-like seeds getting over-dry and rolling out and away in the process.

Coriander is useful for anyone who has a battle with gastric and other symptoms of acidity. Tea can be made from crushed seeds, or seeds can be used in different dishes as flavouring. Thin biscuits made with rice flour, a little Barbados sugar, unsaturated fat and flavoured with Coriander ought not to upset anyone's digestion and might also inhibit the production of too much hydrochloric acid in the digestive juices.

Coriander is one of four herbs, – the others are Liquorice (see page 44), Wormwood and Sage – which are all recommended specially for people who are constantly struggling to increase the alkaline-balance of their systems.

Seeds for growing can usually be obtained from specialist nurseries who sell herb seeds. They can be sown in the autumn and the young plants should over-winter providing the weather is not too harsh, and then flower in the following summer. Once the precious seeds have been gathered (and all herbs must be harvested on warm, still days, preferably in the morning when the dew has dried), they should be dried and then stored in airtight containers.

9.

DILL
(Anethum graveolens)

This tall and handsome herb is not a native of Britain, but it can be grown in gardens in rich soil where it makes a decorative asset to an herbaceous border. It is an umbelliferous plant with rounded umbels of yellow flowers.

Its 'seeds' – which botanically-speaking are its fruits – contain a volatile oil which is something like that of Caraway in flavour. Dill leaves are used as a flavourer for soups, sauces for fish or marrows, cucumber-dressings, or chopped in salads, and they give a most unusual piquancy which the French utilize by adding Dill to their cakes and pastries. In some places the essential oil of Dill was used to scent soaps and perfumes.

Dill has been used as a medicinal herb longer than there have been books in which to describe it. In a tenth-century vocabulary, Alfric, Archbishop of Canterbury, mentions the name as 'Dilla', from the Norse, meaning 'to lull'.

In the sixteenth century Lyte says it was sown in all gardens 'amongst worts and pot-herbs'. The Anglo-Saxon word 'wort', is another old word for a herb or a weed with useful virtues. It often occurs still in popular English plant names like St John's Wort, or St Peter's Wort, which is a country name for Cowslips. Dill is a magic herb which used to be employed to 'keep away the wykked sperytes' and 'Dill, that hindereth witches of their will' is an old English saying.

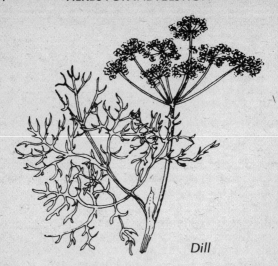

Dill

When church and chapel services, and sermons, were very long people took 'Go to Meeting Seeds' with them to chew and these often included Dill seeds. It is to be hoped that they didn't have the effect of lulling the congregation off to peaceful repose.

Dill-water, of course, is an old remedy to soothe fractious infants; 'for infant flatulence', says a polite Victorian repertory. Culpeper recommended it to 'still the hiccough' and 'to expel the wind and the pains therefrom'.

Five drops of oil of Dill in a little warm water is excellent in cases of discomfort and distension from wind in the stomach, and is still frequently used by some people instead of habit-forming indigestion tablets.

John Evelyn, in his *Acetaria* or *Book about Sallets* in 1680, gives this recipe for 'Dill and Collyflower Pickle': 'Boil the collyflowers till they fall in pieces; then with some of the stalk and the worst of the flower, boil it in a part of the liquer till pretty strong. Then being taken off; strain it and when settled, clean it from the bottom. Then with Dill, gross pepper, a pretty quantity of salt, when cold add as much vinegar as will make it sharp and pour it all upon the Collyflower.' Not, perhaps, ideal for those battling with acid, or too much acid, in the stomach, but good cooks can usually get round the acid-encouraging ingredients in one way or another!

10.

FENNEL
(Foeniculum vulgare)

Fine-leaved Fennel grows wild in plenty of areas near the sea. Its tall, green stems, with their plumes of feathery leaves and umbels of tiny yellow flowers often decorate coastal rural roadsides or cliff tops. It can be sown in gardens, where it will more or less perpetuate itself from wild flower seed. When any part of the plant is pinched it is highly aromatic, the poet John Milton saying that no odour 'more pleased my senses than the smell of sweetest Fennel'.

Fennel has been used since Roman times and probably long before that. It was mentioned in Anglo-Saxon herbals as being used for both culinary and medicinal purposes. The Italian or Florentine Fennel, or *Finocchio*, makes a larger root and can be bought in some greengrocers and cooked (or shredded finely, raw), as a delicious vegetable or salad ingredient.

It is also a useful flavourer for somewhat tasteless vegetables, and improves sauces and soups as long as it is only added in very small quantity. In Victorian days, in parts of Kent, a fishmonger would add a branch of Fennel if a mackerel was ordered. A writer of that period said too that Fennel seeds were boiled and the liquid drunk 'to relieve those who had eaten poisonous mushrooms and other herbs'. It has obviously long had a reputation for absorbing toxic effects, as Culpeper stated that 'One good old custom is

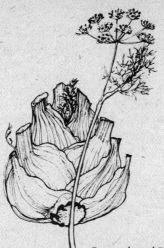

Fennel and Finocchio

not yet left off, viz. to boil Fennel with fish for it consumes the phlegmatic humours which fish most plentifully afford and annoy the body with'. Fennel seed used always to be cooked with conger.

Fennel seeds make a pleasing sweet-substitute, like those of Dill, a habit which must have been indulged in for a very long time for Piers Plowman mentions, 'a Farthynge-worth of Fennel-seed for fastynge days'. They are nice to chew and good for those who suffer from more or less any stomach worries. They are another ingredient of 'Gripe Water'.

Fresh chopped young Fennel leaves infused in milk make a soothing between-meals drink and there are many other old country recipes for the plant's use. Parkinson suggested that 'the roots are used in broths and the leaves more seldom', and 'Cowcumbers and other fruits are pickled in it'. Fennel seeds should be put in 'Pippin Pies' and 'divers other such baked fruits,' as also 'unto bread to give it a better relish'.

A seventeenth-century recipe could still make an unusual dish to-day: 'To make a "Sallet of Fennel", take young Fennel about a span long in the spring, tye it up in bunches as you do Sparragrass: when your skillet boyle, put in enough to make a dish; when it is boiled and drained, dish it up as you do Sparragrass; pour on butter and send it up.'

GENTIAN
(Gentiana lutea)

This yellow-flowered Gentian grows wild in the European mountains and often fills the summer Alpine meadows with a 'sea of gold'. It is sometimes pictured in books about Alpine Flowers, with its whorls of flowers each supported by a pair of broad, leaf-like bracts. It seeds abundantly and germinates fairly easily and it is possible to grow it here in flatter habitats from seeds. It will, however, do best on a chalky soil.

Gerard, the old botanist and herbalist, had plants sent from Burgundy for his garden on Holborn Hill, in London.

It is a most ornamental, colourful and tall plant.

Yellow Gentian was a constituent of 'Stockton Bitters', being used together with the root of Sweet Flag. It is the principal vegetable bitter used in medicine. The root of the plant is used both to flavour a liqueur and as a tonic to alleviate many different stomach symptoms. It should not be taken by sufferers from gastric ulcers before they consult a medical herbalist, as it may not suit certain individuals at all.

Culpeper suggested that 'it strengthens the stomach exceedingly and helps digestions; it preserves the heart and preserves it against fainting and swooning ... and restoreth an appetite to their meat to such as have lost it'. Those who have tasted this yellow-flowered Gentian say that it tastes sweet at first and bitter afterwards.

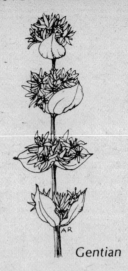

Gentian

Many herbalists, far more modern than Culpeper, stress the value of this large and beautiful herb for medicinal purposes, saying that it is useful in hysteria and for those who complain of vertigo on rising or moving. It is also said particularly to suit people who are better when they are in the fresh air, as well as those who frequently complain of frontal headaches, or 'tender heads'.

Yellow Gentian is prescribed by qualified herbalists at times for sufferers from indigestion who have thick, ropey saliva, acid risings, and a feeling of weight or constant pain in the stomach which is distended and tense. But, as has already been said, it is not a herbal drug for amateurs to prescribe, although it helps such a variety of symptoms, even nausea, if and when it is indicated.

HOPS
(Humulus lupulus)

Hops are not thought to be true native plants in Britain, although the cultivated strains, used for beer-making, have been grown for several centuries here. They form a profitable crop and undoubtedly some have become naturalized and now often appear in our hedgerows.

Hops are climbers and they grow up and pull themselves aloft by the help of stronger-stemmed plants. Pliny said that a hop 'vine', or plant, could kill a willow tree by binding itself tightly round it, but the growth of Hop plants is so attractive and decorative that usually any 'escapes' are much sought by flower-arrangers.

Fields of cultivated Hops need a lot of nourishment. Thomas Tusser, the sixteenth-century agriculturist said: 'Choose soil for the Hop of the rottonest mould, well-doonged and wrought, as a garden plot should be'. Gerard also stressed the plant's needs when he wrote that 'the Hop joyeth in a fruitfull soil'.

The prim Victorians delighted in the scent from Hops, recording that they provided one of summer's loveliest fragrances, together with that of 'Bean fields or blossoming Broom or Briar Roses, or that from fields of Lavender.' It is interesting to hear opinions, but Hops' scent hardly seems to be comparable now with that of the other flowering plants mentioned above.

Hops were brought to Britain from the Low

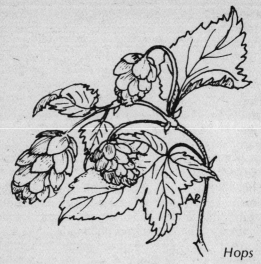

Hops

Countries, or Artois, in the reign of Henry II, but their cultivation may have been restricted later during Henry VI's time, as he mentioned them as these 'wicked weeds called Hops'. The difference between Beer, which had long been a national drink and Ale, was that Ale was said not to be hopped, although plenty of other herbs were included in its brewing.

Hops have many helpful qualities, as well as 'imparting an agreeable and aromative flavour to Beer'; they are soporific (See *Herbs to Help You Sleep*, in this series), and an infusion of Hops makes a good tonic and blood purifier. A modern herbalist maintains that the bitter principle in Hops makes a good tonic for the stomach and digestion and improves the appetite. Because this principle is soothing it can help to break the vicious circle of poor sleep disturbed by mild indigestion, and indigestion caused by sheer exhaustion.

In the old days an infusion of Hop leaves in

sherry was recommended for 'chronic sleeplessness', but the sherry is probably an unnecessary, even if pleasant addition, and an infusion made by pouring boiling water over the Hops would be cheaper and better for anyone suffering from over-acidity.

Hops could almost be said to help sufferers from what is vaguely known as 'nervous indigestion', especially if they have a tendency towards over-excitability. Hops are also said to help those with nausea and dizziness, as well as those who have headaches from hangovers!

The popularity of Hops in the countryside is reflected in the number of country names they have been given over the years, which include 'Sparragrass' (when picked as very young shoots and used as a mock Asparagus); 'Seeders', 'Colegates', 'Whitebines' (as the opposite of 'Blackbines,' or the poisonous Black Bryony); and 'Goldings' for when they are dry and ripe.

13.

LIQUORICE
(Glycyrrhiza glabra)

Liquorice root, *Réglisse* in French, has been known as a multi-purpose herb, including, as Culpeper says, 'all diseases of the breast and lungs', but especially, perhaps, as an ingredient of herbal stomach tonics, through the ages.

Modern herbalists classify it as one of the four best herbs for those who are 'full of acidity', together with Coriander, Sage and Wormwood.

This particular Liquorice, which used to be known as the 'official' *Glycyrrhiza*, is native to Spain and Italy but has been cultivated in Britain since the days of Elizabeth I, when it was taken medicinally and utilized in the brewing of a dark brown malt liquor known as 'porter'. No one appears to know why this drink was thus named unless, as the dictionary suggests, it was as the favourite drink of London porters that it earned its name.

Later, Liquorice was used as an ingredient in the manufacture of sweets which were named after the herb. The most famous Liquorice sweets were the little 'cakes' made at Pontefract in Yorkshire.

Glycyrrhiza glabra is a deep-rooted perennial plant which is best not harvested until it is three years old, when it has obviously formed a strong root. It has a relative in Britain *Astragalus glycyphyllos* growing wild in a few counties, and always sparsely, on chalk. It is called Wild Liquorice here, which shows that once upon a

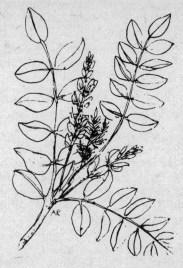

Liquorice

time it too was probably used for the same
purposes as the 'official' member of the botanical
family. In one village in West Sussex this plant
grows on the school wall and because of its rarity
is zealously guarded by the children if botanists or
wild-flowerers come along to have a look at it.

The European Liquorice was mentioned by
Theophrastus, who used it for asthma-sufferers
and to help those who had pain from ulcers.
Modern pharmacognosists have discovered that
the plant is exceptionally rich in calcium and
magnesium.

14

MARSHMALLOW
(Althaea officinalis)

Marshmallow is another mucilaginous plant and one that is famous because of its demulcent healing abilities for different purposes, which will be mentioned later.

First, a little description of this now not very common wild flower which seems to prefer to grow within sight, or at least smell, of the sea. It is found at the top of beaches, sometimes in estuaries, and even far up rivers, when the water is tidal and retains a degree of salinity.

Marshmallow is a tall, velvet-leaved plant, not unlike a hollyhock, to which it is related, with far smaller pale pink flowers that each open for one day only. Its pulped roots and soft, suede-green leaves were once used to make 'Syrup of Marshmallow', which was given to children for many minor winter ills. It was said to 'help them with the cough' and 'all those who suffer from inflammatory conditions of the belly'.

Culpeper says that 'it is an herbe of Venus. The leaves thereof are used to loosen the belly gently.'

The hairy leaves are made into a tea by infusing a few in boiling water, providing a soothing and non-acid drink. Used externally, these leaves make a superb poultice for 'drawing all manner of boyles to a point in order to let out their evil'.

'Marshmallows', of course, those deliciously soft and chewy sweets, were originally made from the roots of the plant, which contain all the

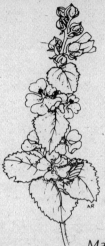

Marshmallow

necessary ingredients in a truly natural form. Nowadays they are made commercially from starches, sugar and gelatine. It is somewhat sad that so many of the old recipes are impracticable in this day and age because of the scarcity of the plants themselves. Conservationists would be horrified if herbally-minded confectioners descended on the few remaining areas where the pretty pale pink-flowered Marshmallows still grow, but it is interesting to know that Britons once, particularly in East Anglia, were able to invent innoxious sweets and make them from a local herb.

15.

MATÉ
(Ilex paraguayensis)

Maté tea – instead of Indian or Ceylon or China tea, all of which contain tannin and some of which are now dyed in order to look a better colour – is thoroughly recommended to all who are conscious of imperfect health.

This South American holly makes history, for Maté-growing has spread to all other tea-growing countries and the harvesting and preparation of its small, somewhat leathery leaves can be arduous.

However the end-product produces an interestingly flavoured drink and one with many benefits to confer. Perhaps the chief is its amazing quality of satisfying the appetite. A cup of Maté is reasonably filling! It is sustaining too and Maté-drinkers are not always rushing off to find snacks between meals.

Many people find that Maté tea is a useful bedtime drink; it certainly has a gently tranquillizing effect on the whole system, which it seems to relax. On the other hand it is equally useful in the day-time and although it tastes very strange at first, one soon becomes almost an addict, for there is much that is pleasant in its smoky flavour.

It is essential that Maté tea is made freshly for each 'sitting'. Unlike some herbal teas, of which enough can be brewed to last a day, Maté goes black if it is kept.

Some Maté-imbibers like a squeeze of lemon in

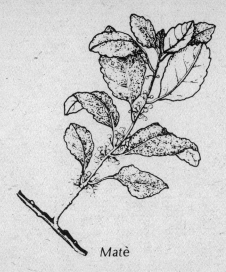

Matè

their drink, others prefer a little honey, but it is best drunk plain for helping those with any difficulty with their alkaline-balance.

It is always rather amusing to read in the older herb books that Maté is one of the herbs which stimulate the intelligence. There are, of course, several others including Bay, with which the Greeks crowned their brilliant men. However, Maté has this attribute, which it may endow upon its followers and it also has a wonderful reputation for helping rheumatic and arthritic victims.

The name Maté was originally given to the pot from which the natives in South America imbibed the infusion. Each 'tea-party' sharing a pot drank the tea through the spout of the pot, called the 'bombilla', which was perforated 'at the top to prevent the swallowing of the pulverised herb'. Travellers were often invited to join in and it is easy to imagine Victorian Britishers and others finding it distasteful. They, so we are told served 'theirs in little glass tubes'!

16

MEADOWSWEET
(Filipendula ulmaria)

Meadowsweet, with its heads of creamy flowers, is one of our most beautiful wild flowers. It is rapidly getting scarcer now that its favourite damp fields, ditches and pond-sides are being drained and the countryside, too, diminishes to make more room for roads, industry and for house-building.

The picture of it growing in plentiful masses of frothy blossom is changing fast since A.M.F. Duclaux wrote, earlier this century:

See the meadowsweet is white against the water-
courses,
Marshy lands are kingcup-gay and bright with streams
and sources.
Dew-bespangled shines the hill, where half-abloom the
gorse is
And all the northern fallow streams beneath the
ploughing horses.

However, there is still some of this delightful wild plant left and it has always been a favourite of country people, who gave it all kinds of pleasing names like 'Bridewort', 'Queen of the Meadows' and 'Dolloff' in the past.

Meadowsweet is a many-purpose herb that has been used in a variety of ways for centuries. It was one of the three most sacred herbs of the Druids; the others being Water Mint and Vervain. Water Mint, of course, like Meadowsweet, was gathered to be trodden underfoot as a strewing herb before carpets were used, and 'Queen Elizabeth of

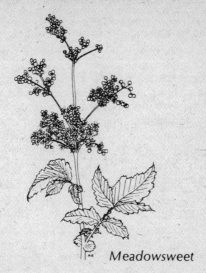

Meadowsweet

famous memory, did more desire it than any other herbe to strew her chambers withall', or so Parkinson said.

Before that we are told how it was used, together with forty-nine other ingredients, in a drink called 'Save', that Chaucer mentions in his *'Knight's Tale'*, and Gerard too, said that 'the floures boiled in wine and drunke, do make the heart merrie'.

There is no need for the wine as Meadowsweet leaves, or flower-heads, fresh or dry, make a wonderful, mild digestive tea for those who need an 'antacid'. It is particularly included here because of this virtue. Meadowsweet has been tried repeatedly in the author's home and has always been a helpful, acid-quenching, as well as thirst-quenching, drink. It is helpful to those with cystitis, or the form of bladder soreness caused by very acid urine, too.

The Victorians delighted in using the flowers as they made them into scented garlands, although they advised very strongly that these garlands should be worn out of doors, the scent from the plant being somewhat heavy and 'deleterious' in a closed room.

What is surprising is the difference between the flowers' scent, which is delicious, and the odour that comes from crushed or broken stems. The latter to some people is reminiscent of disinfectants. But whatever their smell, its roots were supposed to be 'much sought by swine' and cattle browse on the whole plant with apparent pleasure still.

17.

MINT
(Mentha spp.)

There is no doubt at all that Mint is the best known and usually the most available herb to help indigestion, whether it is used as a carminative for mild wind, or for acute distension, or even to soothe inflammation of the membrane of the stomach.

When Tom Hood lay a-dying he turned his eyes feebly towards the window on hearing it rattle in the night: whereupon his wife who was watching him, said softly: 'It's only the wind, dear,' to which last he replied with a ready sense of humour, indomitable to the last: 'Then put a peppermint lozenge on the sill!'

This delightful story was quoted by Dr Fernie, in his *Meals Medicinal*.

Certainly it is Peppermint that is most frequently used, but most of the Mints help to provide a safe relief from unpleasant stomach symptoms.

Peppermint (*Mentha piperita*) is cultivated extensively on the Continent but does not grow well in Britain now. A fungal rust paralyzes it and quickly ruins a crop. Other Mints can be grown more easily here in gardens and are simply propagated by root cuttings. They need to be kept under strict control, or, like Balm, they will soon take over the whole garden.

Tradition has it that England was the first European country to use Mint, and Peppermint is

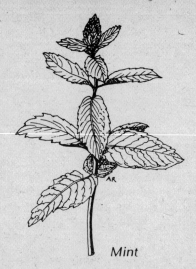

Mint

thought to have appeared as a separate species for the first time when Ray's *Sinopsis Stirpium* was written. It was subsequently named in the London Pharmacoepia of 1721. Nowadays oil of Peppermint could really be named as the most important of all the volatile plant oils in the world.

There are many stories about the properties of Mint. The Druids' sacred Water Mint was gathered by a farmer in the last century on Scalpa in the Hebrides. He had had 'much damage done to his wheat by the depredations of mice', so 'gathered a quantity of Water Mint from a neighbouring brook, placed it among his wheat-sheaves, after which it remained untouched.' Actually, too, a few drops of oil of Peppermint are a good moth-preventive.

But as a medicinal herb Mint is soothing as well as gently stimulating to the whole of the digestive system, and it is comforting to know that Mint is completely safe to use. Mint tea can be made in a variety of strengths, and sipped hot and slowly.

Mint has many culinary uses and can be used as a digestive flavourer chopped up in scrambled eggs, or in mixed herbal sauces or in stuffing for meat, poultry, fish or omelettes. *But* when using raw herbs in this way, do not add them until the last minute when possible, so that their fine flavours are not wholly cooked out.

18

OATS
(Avena sativa)

It is surprising that this wild Oat is such a persistent plant that no weed-killers can eradicate it, without, of course, damaging the cereal crop in which it appears; and that accordingly it still has to be weeded out by hand!

As a medicinal herb, together with Barley and other grains (*see page 17*) it provides a soothing, nerve-quietening effect if infused, strained and drunk at night, before going to bed.

Other – cultivated – Oats have been used as cooked and uncooked grain foods for centuries and tradition has it that the Scots are such a fine, brave, strong and courageous race because so many of them have been brought up on porridge and oatmeal. The latter is even used in their famous Haggis!

Porridge, eaten slowly, with a little milk, not cream, and without any sweetening, makes an excellent breakfast food. If it is made from Oats that have been grown 'organically', that is without the use of artificial fertilizers or weed-killer, the porridge will be better still.

Muesli, with raw crushed, rolled or flaked Oats, grated apples, a little honey, a few sultanas or raisins and even some grated nuts, is also excellent, possibly giving the best start to the day that anyone could ever wish. But it is 'tough' and needs a great deal of mastication and is not a dish to be hurried through. Proper chewing, plenty of

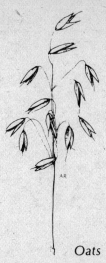

Oats

time in which to eat it appreciatively, complete
lack of anxiety, stress or impatience, are all
needed if it is to be digested well. This goes for all
eating, of course, especially for those with tender
tummies.

If breakfast has to be rushed, or eaten in an
atmosphere full of tenseness, Slippery Elm, made
like a smooth, thin porridge (*see page 61*) is better
than Oats in any form.

It is curious, returning to wild Oats, that they
usually help harassed women more than harassed
men! There seems to be no easily understandable
reason and it probably lies in some hormonal
activity undiscovered so far in the plant's make-up.
However, for women, wild Oat tea can make an
excellent tonic after debilitating diseases when the
digestion is weak. It may also, if used in tincture
form and a few drops in water taken instead of a
tisane, be good for ridding the stomach of catarrh.
A few drops of this tincture makes a helpful pick-
me-up too for those who are nervously exhausted

and if taken regularly will be found to help concentration or, as someone else put it, will 'strengthen the ability to keep the mind on one subject at a time'; a most useful asset for those with excitable 'grass-hopper' minds!

19

PASSION-FLOWER
(Passiflora incarnata)

The rosy Passion-flower grows in warm areas of America and in the West Indies, where its fruits are known as 'May-bobs' or 'May-apples', which – according to Johnson's edition of Gerard's *Herbal* – were called 'Granadillas' by the Spaniards in the West Indies, and 'Maracoes' by the Virginians.

There are, of course, more familiar Passion-flowers to us, here in Britain. We can grow the beautiful, somewhat fantastic flowers of the Blue Passion-flower up walls, providing they are sheltered, and we can also grow the Edible Passion-flower fruit (*Passiflora edulis*) under glass.

Neither of these *Passiflora* unfortunately give the same therapeutic virtues as the American herb.

Passiflora incarnata is included here, not as a digestive or as a demulcent, soothing herb for the stomach, but because it is a safe, non-habit-forming, harmless tranquillizer. It is often, indeed, used with Skullcap, another wonderfully quietening herb, and either separately or together (your medical herbalist's advice should be sought in this matter) they can give a hard-working mind a lot of peace and rest by helping to ameliorate the physical results of nervous exhaustion.

This rosy Passion-flower, as well as producing easy, dreamless sleep, will soothe a troublesome night cough and is a herb very well worth trying at

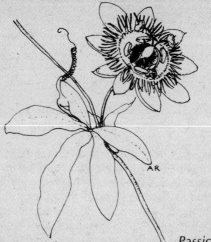

Passion-flower

the start of a campaign to get rid of acidity and its
unpleasant effects on the physical system.

It is interesting to know why these flowers were
christened 'Passion-flowers'. If you look carefully
at the picture you can just see the flower's strange
'arrangements' of the sepals, corona, anthers and
stigmas. These are much easier to see in a live
flower, but they were said to represent, according
to Spanish friars, 'The Passion of our Saviour'.
Starting in the middle of the flower, the three
stigmas were thought to look like three nails; the
five anthers marked the five wounds. The spiky
corona stood for the crown of thorns and the ten
sepals were the ten apostles, without Peter, who
denied Him, and Judas, who betrayed Him. The
coiled tendrils even suggested the scourging
whips that were used at the time of the
Crucifixion.

20

SLIPPERY ELM
(Ulmus fulva)

Slippery Elm, Red Elm, Indian Elm and Moose Elm are all names in America and Canada for a small, very valuable Elm tree that is much sought after for its inner bark. It grows wild along the banks of streams with Swamp Oaks, Red Maples and Hackberry plants, but it can also be found – although it grows even smaller in such dry situations – on rocky ridges.

The bark, which is fragrant on drying, is rough and grey and very useful for a variety of medicinal purposes. The discovery of a tree, unfortunately, often led to its destruction, as it was literally skinned alive just for its mucilaginous inner bark.

Trees are actually cultivated on purpose for their bark and left alone until they are about ten years old; then they are cut down, so that this precious bark can be stripped off.

Slippery Elm is an official drug of the U.S. Pharmacoepia (1931) and is an important crop, as the dried bark forms a highly nutritious, easily assimilable food after it has been powdered and prepared for use.

It is most easily made into a smooth gruel and can be bought for this purpose, sometimes with milk powder or malt already added to make it more palatable. Nutritionists say that the demulcent, soothing food exerts a protective influence on the whole of the digestive tract when the latter is inflamed.

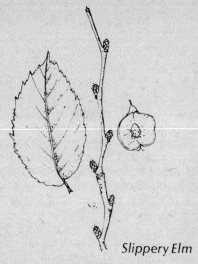

Slippery Elm

Certainly, the thin gruel makes an easy breakfast or supper for anyone who is in a rush, or who is tired at night. It is splendid for convalescents as well and for those who do not fancy food but who need some light nourishment. There are no other similar foods that are anything like as good, because of the healing virtues of the Slippery Elm itself.

Taken in this way Slippery Elm makes an indispensable part of the diet for those who suffer from acidity, or the inability to keep other foods down, or with an irritated, sore stomach. Its value cannot be over-stressed for those who suffer from stomach pain.

It is perfectly possible to sweeten it, or to have cream with it, but neither is necessary, and for those of 'weak digestive ability' it is better made with half milk and half water, without anything else added to it at all.

THERAPEUTIC INDEX

Antacid Teas, Balm, Barley Water, Brown Rice, Celery, Coriander, Gentian, Hops, Liquorice, Marshmallow.

Breath-cleanser, Agrimony.

Carminative, *See* **'Wind'**

Demulcent, *See* **'Soothing herbs'**

Depression, Balm, Celery.

Excitability, Hops, Oats, Passion-flower.

Exhaustion, Oats, Passion-flower.

Headache, Gentian, Hops.

Heartburn, Celery, Chamomile.

Hiccoughs, Dill.

Irritability, Chamomile.

Mental Stimulation, Balm, Maté, Oats.

Mucilaginous herbs, Comfrey, Marshmallow, Slippery Elm.

Nausea, Chamomile, Gentian, Hops.

Restlessness, Hops, Maté, Oats, Passion-flower.

Rheumatism, Agrimony, Maté.

Ropey Saliva, Gentian.

Seeds to chew, Celery, Dill, Fennel.

Sleeplessness, Celery, Chamomile, Dill, Hops, Oats, Passion-flower.

Soothing herbs, Comfrey, Marshmallow, Passion-flower, Slippery Elm.

Stomach tonic, Agrimony, Chamomile, Hops, Liquorice, Oats.

Wind, Balm, Chamomile, Dill, Mint.

everybody's home herbal

HERBS AND FRUIT FOR SLIMMERS

Ceres. *Illustrated.* Explains how some herbs can help to get rid of superfluous flesh and also—if they are taken with the various fruits of the earth, like grapefruit, avocado pears, tomatoes, peppers and mushrooms—how they can even help to prevent the formation of unwanted layers of fat. Slimming (or anti-fat) herbs can be taken in the pleasant form of teas or tisanes and they work in a variety of ways. Author gives instructions on how these are made. *Contents include:* Blue Flag; Borage; Fennel; Juniper; Maté tea; Parsley and other raw flavourers; Rose Geranium and other cooking flavourers.

HERBS FOR HEADACHES AND MIGRAINE

Nalda Gosling FNIMH, MBNOA, ND, DO. A practising medical herbalist, naturopath and osteopath—and President of the National Institute of Medical Herbalists—explains the causes of headaches, devoting a whole chapter to migraine, and sets out dietetic measures to take along with the chosen selection of twenty-one herbs that have proved helpful in relieving these distressing and incapacitating complaints.

The effectiveness of herbal remedies has been proved by long usage and research, and such treatment aims at removing the cause rather than just the symptoms—a much more satisfactory approach than that of taking aspirin and other pain-relieving drugs which afford only temporary relief and carry the risk of side-effects.

HERBS FOR RHEUMATISM AND ARTHRITIS

Sarah Beckett. Herbs cleanse the whole system and are therefore ideal for treating rheumatic conditions. This book describes twenty-five herbs for the treatment of muscular rheumatism (which includes fibrositis) and rheumatism of the joints, or arthritis (which includes osteo and rheumatoid arthritis and gout). The herbs featured help rid the body of excess acids, purify the blood, and soothe the aches and pains of muscles and bones. The intake of correct food plays a very important part in the treatment of rheumatic diseases and author provides supplementary advice on dietetics, vitamin therapy, Epsom salts baths, exercise and relaxation techniques.

HERBS FOR THE HEART AND CIRCULATION

THE NUTRITIONAL APPROACH TO CARDIOVASCULAR DISEASE

Nalda Gosling, N.D., D.O. *Illustrated.* Correct nutrition is the key to preventing and curing heart disease! Cardiovascular disease in the West kills more people than all other diseases put together. In England and Wales a 12% rise in circulatory deaths was recorded for 1951-1973. Here over twenty herbs are described which benefit heart conditions and contributory symptoms. Full details on how to take each herb (infusion, tablets, etc.), and precise directions as to dosage.